NALTREXONE

DANIEL GARCIA

What is naltrexone?

Naltrexone is a physician recommended medicine used to treat liquor use jumble and narcotic use problem. It assists you with halting utilizing these substances and stay off them.

Naltrexone has a place with a class of medications known as narcotic bad guys and works by obstructing the mu narcotic receptor. It impedes the impacts of liquor and narcotic meds, forestalling the inebriation these substances cause. Naltrexone likewise changes how the nerve center, pituitary organ and adrenal organ (hypothalamic-pituitary-adrenal pivot, HPA hub) collaborate to smother how much liquor consumed.

Naltrexone comes as a drawn out discharge intramuscular infusion (Vivitrol) and as oral tablets. The marked adaptations of naltrexone tablets (Revia, Depade) have been stopped, however conventional variants are accessible.

Naltrexone tablets were first supported by the US Food and Medication Organization (FDA) in 1984. In 2006, the FDA additionally endorsed Vivitrol, the drawn out discharge intramuscular infusion type of naltrexone.

What is naltrexone utilized for?

Naltrexone is a physician recommended drug that is utilized:

to treat liquor reliance

for the bar of the impacts of exogenously regulated narcotics. To forestall backslide to narcotic reliance, after narcotic detoxification.

You ought to quit drinking liquor or utilizing narcotics prior to beginning naltrexone.

Naltrexone hydrochloride ought not be utilized in youngsters and youths under 18 years.

Significant data

Naltrexone can cause serious incidental effects, including:

1. Chance of narcotic excess.

You can unintentionally go too far in two ways.

Naltrexone hinders the impacts of narcotic medications. Try not to take a lot of narcotics, including narcotic containing meds, like heroin or solution torment pills, to attempt to defeat the narcotic hindering impacts of this medicine. This can prompt serious injury, unconsciousness, or demise.

After you get a portion of the drawn out discharge infusion type of this medicine, its impeding impact gradually diminishes and totally disappears after some time. Assuming you have utilized narcotic road drugs or narcotic containing meds previously, utilizing narcotics in sums that you utilized before treatment can prompt excess and passing. You may likewise be more delicate with the impacts of lower measures of narcotics:

after you have gone through detoxification

at the point when your next naltrexone infusion is expected

on the off chance that you miss a portion of this prescription

after you stop naltrexone treatment

You must tell your family and individuals nearest to you of this expanded aversion to narcotics and the gamble of excess.

You or somebody near you ought to call 911 or move crisis clinical assistance immediately in the event that you:

experience difficulty relaxing

turn out to be exceptionally sleepy with eased back relaxing

have slow, shallow breathing (little chest development with relaxing) feel faint, extremely lightheaded, confounded, or have strange side effects

Converse with your medical services supplier about naloxone, a medication that is accessible to patients for the crisis therapy of a narcotic excess.

Call 911 or move crisis clinical assist with correcting away in all instances of known or thought narcotic excess, regardless of whether naloxone is directed.

Extreme responses at the site of the naltrexone infusion (infusion site responses).

Certain individuals have had extreme infusion site responses, including tissue passing (putrefaction), while getting naltrexone infusions. A portion of these infusion site responses have required a medical procedure. This prescription should be infused by a medical care supplier. Summon your medical care supplier right assuming you notice any of the accompanying at any of your infusion destinations:

serious torment

the region feels hard

huge area of enlarging

protuberances

rankles

a fresh injury

a dull scab

Inform your medical services supplier regarding any response at an infusion site that concerns you, deteriorates over the long haul, or gets worse by about fourteen days after the infusion.

3. Abrupt narcotic withdrawal.

Any individual who gets naltrexone should not utilize any kind of narcotic (should be sans narcotic) including road drugs, remedy torment meds, hack, cold, or loose bowels meds that contain narcotics, or narcotic reliance medicines, buprenorphine or methadone, for no less than 7 to 14 days prior to beginning this prescription. Utilizing narcotics in the 7 to 14 days before you begin getting treatment might make you abruptly have side effects of narcotic withdrawal when you get treatment. Abrupt narcotic withdrawal can be serious, and you might have to go to the medical clinic.

You should be without narcotic prior to getting naltrexone except if your medical services supplier concludes that you don't have to go through detox first. All things considered, your PCP might choose to give this drug in a clinical office that can treat you for unexpected narcotic withdrawal.

4. Liver harm or hepatitis. Naltrexone can cause liver harm or hepatitis.

Let your medical care supplier know if you have any of the accompanying side effects of liver issues during therapy with this medicine:

stomach region torment enduring in excess of a couple of days

dim pee

yellowing of the whites of your eyes

sleepiness

Your medical services supplier might have to quit treating you with this prescription on the off chance that you get signs or side effects of a serious liver issue.

You should illuminate each specialist that treats you that you are taking Naltrexone. Non-narcotic based sedatives ought to be utilized in the event that you require a sedative in a crisis circumstance. Assuming you need to utilize narcotic containing sedatives, you might require higher dosages than expected. You may likewise be more delicate to the secondary effects (breathing hardships and circulatory issues).

Who shouldn't utilize naltrexone?

Try not to utilize naltrexone if you:

are utilizing or have an actual reliance on/dependence on narcotic containing medications or narcotic road drugs.

To see whether you have an actual reliance on narcotics, your medical services supplier might provide you with a little infusion of a medication called naloxone. This is known as a naloxone challenge test. Assuming you get side effects of narcotic withdrawal after the naloxone challenge test, don't begin treatment with naltrexone around then. Your medical services supplier might rehash the test after you have quit utilizing narcotics to see whether beginning this medication is protected.

are having narcotic withdrawal side effects. Narcotic withdrawal side effects might happen when you have been taking narcotics routinely and afterward stop.

Side effects of narcotic withdrawal might include:

nervousness

restlessness

yawning

fever

perspiring

weepy eyes

runny nose

goose pimples

precariousness

hot or cold flushes

muscle throbs

muscle jerks

anxiety

queasiness and heaving

the runs

stomach cramps

Let your medical services supplier know if you have any of these side effects prior to taking this medicine.

are taking methadone

have serious liver issues or intense hepatitis

have extreme kidney issues

are susceptible to naltrexone or any of the fixings in the detailing of it you use or the fluid used to blend the injectable structure (diluent). See underneath for a total rundown of fixings.

What would it be a good idea for me to tell my PCP prior to utilizing naltrexone?

Before you get naltrexone, let your medical care supplier know if you:

have liver issues

use or misuse road (unlawful) drugs

have hemophilia or other draining issues

have kidney issues

have some other ailments

have liquor reliance and use narcotics

How could I utilize naltrexone?

Utilizing narcotics in the 7 to 14 days before you begin getting naltrexone might make you unexpectedly have side effects of narcotic withdrawal. To keep away from this, you shouldn't utilize narcotics for at least 7-10 days prior to beginning treatment with naltrexone.

Step by step instructions to take naltrexone tablets

Continuously take this medication precisely as your primary care physician has told you. Check with your primary care physician or drug specialist in the event that you are don't know.

Take this drug once a day by mouth as your PCP tells you to.

How much time you ought to take this prescription for will be chosen by your PCP. The typical length of treatment is three months. Be that as it may, in specific cases, a more extended time of treatment might be valuable.

How you will get a naltrexone infusion

Your infusion will be given by a medical services supplier, around 1 time every month.

Try not to endeavor to infuse yourself with this drug. Serious responses, some that might require hospitalization, could occur.

Naltrexone is given as an infusion into a muscle in your backside utilizing an exceptional needle that accompanies it.

After this medicine is infused, it goes on for a month and it can't be taken out from the body.

Whenever you want clinical treatment, make certain to tell the treating medical services supplier that you are getting this drug and notice when you triumphed ultimately your last portion. This is significant in light of the fact that naltrexone can likewise impede the impacts of narcotic containing meds that may be endorsed for you for torment, hack or colds, or looseness of the bowels.

Convey composed data with you consistently to alarm medical services suppliers that you are taking this medicine so they can treat you appropriately in a crisis. Ask your medical services supplier how you can get a wallet card to convey with you.

What occurs in the event that I miss a portion?

On the off chance that you neglect to take your naltrexone tablet, accept it as quickly as time permits. Notwithstanding, assuming it is nearly time for your next portion, avoid the missed portion and return to your ordinary dosing plan. Try not to take a twofold portion to compensate for a neglected portion.

What occurs on the off chance that I glut?

Assuming you take more naltrexone tablets than you ought to, tell your Primary care physician or Drug specialist or contact your closest clinic crisis office right away.

What would it be a good idea for me to keep away from while utilizing naltrexone?

Try not to drive a vehicle, work hardware, or do other risky exercises until you have at least some idea what this medicine means for you. Naltrexone might cause you to feel discombobulated and languid.

Dosing data

Tablets:

Liquor addiction: The suggested portion is 1 tablet (50 mg) one time per day

Narcotic reliance: Begin with a portion of a tablet (25 mg) and on the off chance that no withdrawal signs happen increment to the portion to 1 tablet (50 mg) a day from that point on

Intramuscular infusion:

The suggested portion is naltrexone 380 mg conveyed intramuscularly (IM) as a gluteal infusion, at regular intervals or one time per month, rotating bum for each ensuing.

What are the symptoms of naltrexone?

Serious symptoms of naltrexone include:

See 'Significant data' above

Discouraged mind-set. Here and there this prompts self destruction, or self-destructive considerations, and self-destructive way of behaving. Tell your relatives and individuals nearest to you that you are taking this prescription.

You, a relative, or individuals nearest to you ought to summon your medical services supplier right in the event that you become discouraged or have any of the accompanying side effects of melancholy, particularly on the off chance that they are new, more terrible, or concern you:

You feel miserable or have crying spells.

You are not generally keen on seeing your companions or doing things you used to appreciate.

You are resting much more or significantly not exactly expected.

You feel irredeemable or defenseless.

You are crabbier, furious, or forceful than expected.

You are pretty much hungry than expected or notice a major change in your body weight.

You experience difficulty focusing.

You feel drained or languid constantly.

You have considerations about harming yourself or taking your life.

You have visualizations.

Pneumonia. Certain individuals getting this treatment have had a particular kind of pneumonia that is brought about by an unfavorably susceptible response. Assuming that this happens to you, your might should be treated in the medical clinic. Tell your medical care supplier immediately assuming that you have any of these side effects during therapy with naltrexone:

windedness or wheezing

hacking that doesn't disappear

Serious unfavorably susceptible responses. Serious unfavorably susceptible responses can occur during or not long after an infusion of naltrexone. Tell your medical care supplier or move clinical assistance immediately in the event that you have any of these side effects of a serious hypersensitive response.

skin rash

enlarging of your face, eyes, mouth, or tongue

inconvenience breathing or wheezing

chest torment

feeling mixed up or swoon

Normal results of naltrexone include:

sickness. Sickness might happen when you initially start this drug, however it can further develop additional time.

regurgitating

drowsiness

uneasiness

cerebral pain

fretfulness

anxiety

stomach torment

difficult joints

muscle torment and muscle cramps

shortcoming

diminished hunger

heart palpitations

expanded pulse

ECG changes

ibido messes

thirst

unsteadiness

increment tear emission

chest torment

loose bowels

clogging

rash

postponed discharge and erectile brokenness

expanded energy

peevishness

expanded perspiring

emotional problems

cold side effects

inconvenience dozing

toothache

Connections

Educate your medical care supplier concerning every one of the meds you take, including remedy and non-professionally prescribed prescriptions, nutrients, and home grown supplements.

Particularly let your medical services supplier know if you take any narcotic containing drugs for agony, hack or colds, or loose bowels.

Assuming you are being treated for liquor reliance yet additionally use or are dependent on narcotic containing medications or narcotic road drugs, you genuinely should advise your medical care supplier prior to beginning naltrexone to try not to have unexpected narcotic withdrawal side effects when you start therapy.

Pregnancy and breastfeeding

Let your primary care physician know if you are pregnant or want to become pregnant. It isn't known whether naltrexone will hurt your unborn child. This prescription ought to possibly be utilized during pregnancy on the off chance that the potential advantages legitimizes the expected gamble to the embryo.

Let your primary care physician know if you are breastfeeding. It isn't known whether naltrexone passes into your milk when it is regulated by IM infusion, and it isn't known whether it can hurt your child. Naltrexone from tablets passes into bosom milk. Converse with your medical services supplier about whether you will breastfeed or take this drug. You shouldn't do both.

Capacity

Store naltrexone tablets at 20° to 25°C.

Store the whole container containing a naltrexone infusion in the cooler (2 °C to 8 °C, 36 °F to 46 °F).

Unrefrigerated, naltrexone microspheres can be put away at temperatures not surpassing 25 °C (77 °F) for close to 7 days preceding organization. Try not to open unrefrigerated item to temperatures over 25 °C (77 °F). Try not to freeze.

Keep hidden and reach of kids.

What are the fixings in naltrexone?

Dynamic fixing: naltrexone (infusion), naltrexone hydrochloride (tablets)

Dormant fixings:

Vivitrol brand infusion: polylactide-co-glycolide (PLG). Diluent fixings: carboxymethylcellulose sodium, polysorbate 20, sodium chloride, sodium hydroxide and hydrochloric corrosive as pH agents, in water for infusion.

Tablets (Chartwell): lactose monohydrate, hypromellose, magnesium stearate, polyethylene glycol, titanium dioxide, colloidal silicon dioxide, hydroxypropyl cellulose, yellow ferric oxide and red ferric oxide.

Latent fixings fluctuate among the different nonexclusive tablet plans of naltrexone. Check the item name for your specific plan for a total rundown of dormant fixings.

The Vivitrol brand of naltrexone infusion is produced and promoted by Alkermes, Inc. 852 Winter Road, Waltham, Mama 02451-1420.

Various organizations assembling and market nonexclusive tablet plans of this prescription.

Know the meds you take. Keep a rundown of them to show your medical services supplier and drug specialist when you get another medication.

For what reason is this prescription recommended?

Naltrexone is utilized alongside directing and social help to assist with peopling who have quit drinking liquor and utilizing road drugs keep on trying not to drink or utilizing drugs. Naltrexone ought not be utilized to treat individuals who are as yet utilizing road medications or drinking a lot of liquor. Naltrexone is in a class of drugs called narcotic bad guys. It works by diminishing the desire for liquor and hindering the impacts of sedative meds and narcotic road drugs.

How might this medication be utilized?

Naltrexone comes as a tablet to take by mouth either at home or under management in a facility or treatment focus. At the point when naltrexone is taken at home, it is typically required once every day regardless of food. At the point when naltrexone is taken in a facility or treatment focus, it could be required one time each day, when each and every other day, when each third day, or when consistently with the exception of Sunday. Follow the bearings on your medicine mark cautiously, and ask your PCP or drug specialist to make sense of any part you don't have the foggiest idea. Take naltrexone precisely as coordinated. Try not to take pretty much of it or take it more frequently than recommended by your primary care physician.

Naltrexone is just useful when it is utilized as a component of a compulsion treatment program. You must go to all guiding meetings, support bunch gatherings, schooling programs, or different medicines suggested by your PCP.

Naltrexone will assist you with trying not to utilize medications and liquor, yet it won't forestall or alleviate the withdrawal side effects that might happen when you quit utilizing these substances. All things considered, naltrexone might cause or deteriorate withdrawal side effects. You shouldn't accept naltrexone on the off chance that you have as of late quit utilizing narcotic prescriptions or narcotic road sedates and are presently encountering withdrawal side effects.

Naltrexone will assist you with keeping away from medications and liquor just for however long you are taking it. Keep on taking naltrexone regardless of whether you feel great. Try not to quit taking naltrexone without conversing with your PCP.

Different purposes for this medication

This medicine might be once in a while endorsed for different purposes; ask your primary care physician or drug specialist for more data.

What exceptional precautionary measures would it be a good idea for me to follow?

Prior to taking naltrexone,

let your PCP and drug specialist know if you are hypersensitive to naltrexone naloxone, other narcotic meds, or some other meds.

let your PCP know if you are taking any narcotic (opiate) meds or road drugs including levomethadyl acetic acid derivation (LAAM, ORLAAM) (not accessible in the US), or methadone (Dolophine, Methadose); and certain meds for the runs, hack, or agony. Additionally, let your PCP know if you have taken any of these meds in the beyond 7 to 10 days. Inquire as to whether you are don't know whether a medicine you have taken is a narcotic. Your primary care physician might arrange specific tests to check whether you have taken any narcotic prescriptions or utilized any narcotic road drugs during the beyond 7 to 10 days. Your PCP will tell you not to take naltrexone in the event that you have taken or utilized narcotics in the beyond 7 to 10 days.

try not to take any narcotic meds or use narcotic road drugs during your treatment with naltrexone. Naltrexone obstructs the impacts of narcotic prescriptions and narcotic road drugs. You may not feel the impacts of these substances assuming that you take or use them at low or typical portions. Assuming you take or utilize higher portions of narcotic prescriptions or medications during your treatment with naltrexone, it might cause serious injury, extreme lethargies (dependable oblivious state), or demise.

you ought to know that assuming you took narcotic drugs before your treatment with naltrexone, you might be more delicate with the impacts of these meds after you finish your treatment. After you finish your treatment, let any specialist know who might endorse meds for you that you were recently treated with naltrexone.

let your PCP know what other remedy and nonprescription prescriptions, nutrients, dietary enhancements, and natural items you are taking or plan to take. Make certain to specify disulfiram (Antabuse) and thioridazine. Your PCP might have to change the portions of your drugs or screen you cautiously for secondary effects.

let your primary care physician know if you have or have at any point had misery or kidney sickness.

let your primary care physician know if you are pregnant, plan to become pregnant, or are bosom taking care of. On the off chance that you become pregnant while taking naltrexone, call your primary care physician.

assuming you really want clinical treatment or medical procedure, including dental medical procedure, tell the specialist or dental specialist that you are taking naltrexone. Wear or convey clinical recognizable proof so medical care suppliers who treat you in a crisis will realize that you are taking naltrexone.

you ought to realize that individuals who abuse medications or liquor frequently become discouraged and some of the time attempt to damage or commit suicide. Getting naltrexone doesn't diminish the gamble that you will attempt to hurt yourself. You or your family ought to summon the specialist right in the event that you experience side effects of wretchedness like sensations of misery, nervousness, sadness, culpability, uselessness, or vulnerability, or contemplating hurting or committing suicide or arranging or attempting to do as such. Be certain that your family knows which side effects might be serious so they can summon the specialist right assuming you can't look for treatment all alone.

What extraordinary dietary guidelines would it be a good idea for me to follow?

Except if your primary care physician tells you in any case, proceed with your ordinary eating regimen.

How would it be a good idea for me to respond on the off chance that I fail to remember a portion?

Accept the missed portion when you recollect it. Notwithstanding, on the off chance that it is nearly time for your next portion, skirt the missed portion and proceed with your normal dosing plan. Try not to take a twofold portion to compensate for a missed one.

What aftereffects might this prescription at any point cause?

Naltrexone might cause aftereffects. Let your primary care physician know if any of these side effects are extreme or don't disappear:

sickness

heaving

stomach torment or squeezing

looseness of the bowels

clogging

loss of hunger

cerebral pain

wooziness

tension

anxiety

touchiness

sorrow

trouble falling or staying unconscious

expanded or diminished energy

sluggishness

muscle or joint torment

rash

A few incidental effects can be serious. Assuming you experience any of these side effects or those recorded in the Significant Advance notice area, call your primary care physician right away:

disarray

mind flights (seeing things or hearing voices that don't exist)

obscured vision

extreme heaving or potentially looseness of the bowels

Naltrexone might cause opposite aftereffects. Call your primary care physician assuming you have any uncommon issues while taking this medicine.

On the off chance that you experience a serious incidental effect, you or your primary care physician might send a report to the Food and Medication Organization's (FDA) MedWatch Unfavorable Occasion Revealing system on the web (http://www.fda.gov/Wellbeing/MedWatch) or by telephone (1-800-332-1088).

What would it be a good idea for me to be familiar with stockpiling and removal of this prescription?

Keep this medicine in the compartment it came in, firmly shut, and far away from kids. Store it at room temperature and away from overabundance intensity and dampness (not in the washroom).

What to stay away from while taking naltrexone?

You shouldn't utilize naltrexone treatment if:

You are getting narcotic (opiate) analgesics.

Assuming you are reliant (dependent) on narcotics.

Assuming you are in an intense narcotic withdrawal or have any side effects of narcotic withdrawal.

In the event that you have bombed a naloxone challenge test or have a positive pee screen for narcotics.

You have intense hepatitis or hepatic disappointment.

In the event that you are unfavorably susceptible or have had an extreme touchiness response to naltrexone, polylactide-co-glycolide (PLG), or some other diluent or idle fixing in the item.

Tell your PCP or other medical care supplier of any new utilization of narcotics or any set of experiences of narcotic reliance prior to beginning naltrexone to try not to have a narcotic withdrawal. Your PCP might expect that you breeze through a naloxone challenge assessment as well as a pee screen for narcotics before naltrexone use.

What is naltrexone utilized for?

Naltrexone is an unadulterated narcotic bad guy supported to treat patients with narcotic use problem (OUD) or liquor use jumble, alongside a restoratively regulated change in behavior patterns program.

Naltrexone itself won't cause opiate like impacts or reliance.

Naltrexone blocks euphoric activities just (meaning it can't prompt compulsion or a "high"). It likewise may hinder the "high" feeling that might make you need to drink liquor. Naltrexone isn't a remedy for dependence on narcotics or liquor.

It is accessible by solution as a long-acting intramuscular infusion (brand name: Vivitrol) or as a 50 mg oral tablet (a conventional).

Naltrexone treatment is begun after you are at this point not subject to narcotics. Naltrexone use for either narcotic use issue or liquor use confusion can prompt withdrawal side effects on the off chance that you are as yet utilizing opiates (narcotics).

Naltrexone ought not be utilized before you complete a therapeutically directed narcotic withdrawal enduring no less than 7 to 14 days. This will assist you with staying away from a narcotic withdrawal that might require hospitalization. In the event that you have been utilizing an all the lengthier acting narcotic like methadone or buprenorphine, your detoxification period might should be longer.

Which narcotics would it be a good idea for me to keep away from with naltrexone?

Individuals utilizing naltrexone shouldn't:

utilize ANY narcotic (for instance: heroin, morphine, codeine, oxycodone, tramadol, hydrocodone or other remedy or unlawful narcotics)

utilize illegal medications

drink liquor

take CNS depressants like narcotics, sedatives, or different medications.

Assuming you endeavor to self-control narcotics, in little portions while on naltrexone, you won't see any impact. Naltrexone obstructs the euphoric and narcotic impacts of the manhandled drug and forestalls sensations of happiness ("high").

Nonetheless, utilizing huge dosages of any narcotic to attempt to sidestep the narcotic hindering impact of naltrexone might prompt serious injury, go too far, extreme lethargies, or demise. You might be more delicate to more modest portions of narcotics once you quit utilizing them, so taking any portion of a narcotic can be risky.

Consider the possibility that I miss a portion of naltrexone.

Miss no portion of naltrexone as endorsed by your primary care physician. Your degree of narcotic resilience will diminish while taking naltrexone.

Past narcotic measurements you utilized preceding naltrexone treatment may now have hazardous results, including discouraged or quit breathing, circulatory breakdown, and passing.

You are likewise helpless against a possibly lethal excess toward the finish of a dosing stretch, in the wake of missing a portion, or subsequent to halting treatment.

On the off chance that you miss taking your oral naltrexone tablet, accept the missed portion when you recollect. Avoid the missed portion assuming it is nearly time for your next booked portion. Try not to take additional medication to make up the missed portion.

On the off chance that you miss your naltrexone infusion arrangement, contact your PCP's office quickly to reschedule one more arrangement at the earliest opportunity.

Consider the possibility that I take an excessive amount of naltrexone.

Adhere to your primary care physician's guidance precisely. The gamble of liver injury is higher with single oral naltrexone portions over 50 mg.

Naltrexone won't cause rapture or a "high". Individuals don't regularly manhandle this medication to incite elation.

Be that as it may, taking an excessive amount of naltrexone might prompt serious liver (hepatic) injury.

Quit taking naltrexone and contact your primary care physician right away assuming you foster stomach torment, white stools, dim pee, or yellowing in the whites of your eyes, all indications of liver injury.

Assuming you have intense hepatitis or other extreme liver illness, you shouldn't utilize naltrexone.

Naltrexone use ought to be kept away from in individuals who are at present utilizing narcotics, in individuals with specific kinds of liver illness or with persistent agony who depend on narcotics for torment control.

Never give or offer naltrexone to any other individual, particularly somebody who is utilizing narcotics. Naltrexone will cause withdrawal side effects in individuals who are utilizing narcotics.

Naltrexone Use and Liquor Reliance

Naltrexone hinders the euphoric impacts and sensations of inebriation from liquor (the "buzz"). This permits individuals with liquor use turmoil to diminish their drinking ways of behaving to the point of staying persuaded to remain in treatment, keep away from backslides, and take drugs.

In any case, naltrexone won't keep you from becoming impeded while drinking liquor. Try not to endeavor to utilize naltrexone so you can drive or perform different exercises affected by liquor.

For the treatment of liquor reliance, you ought not be effectively drinking at the time you start naltrexone treatment. You ought to have the option to keep away from liquor in a short term setting (for instance: at home, work and locally) before commencement of treatment with naltrexone.

You ought to involve naltrexone as a component of a treatment program that incorporates guiding, support gatherings, and other social techniques as suggested by your PCP, for both liquor use jumble and narcotic use issue.

Who can utilize naltrexone?

Naltrexone is endorsed for use in grown-ups 18 years old and more seasoned.

Its utilization in patients more youthful than age 18 has not been endorsed by the FDA. It isn't known whether it is protected and successful in kids under 18 years old.

Naltrexone can be recommended by any medical services proficient who is authorized to endorse drugs. It comes as a tablet (nonexclusive) and long-acting infusion (Vivitrol). The tablets might be managed regardless of food. Organization with food or after feasts might assist with diminishing any stomach incidental effects.

Injectable naltrexone is just given by a medical care supplier. The infusion will be transported straightforwardly to your PCP and you will get the infusion at their office.

Try not to endeavor to provide yourself with an infusion of naltrexone. Injectable naltrexone has been related with serious infusion site issues and skin responses. In the event that you experience any of these responses after a naltrexone infusion, contact your primary care physician right away

Extraordinary agony

Rankles

The region feels hard

Painful injury

Enormous areas of expanding

Dim scab

Knots

Let your primary care physician know if you have kidney (renal) infection before you start naltrexone treatment. Additional watchfulness might be required when you get naltrexone.

On the off chance that you have draining issues, low blood platelets, or a lung condition, tell your PCP before you start naltrexone treatment.

Naltrexone can cause despondency in certain patients. Let your primary care physician know if you have a past filled with despondency, endeavored self-destruction, or other psychological wellness problems before you start naltrexone treatment. Tell your relatives or others near you that you are taking naltrexone. They ought to summon a specialist right in the event that you become discouraged or experience side effects of gloom.

Try not to drive, work large equipment or play out any perilous exercises until you know what naltrexone will mean for you. Naltrexone might make tipsiness and sluggishness and influence your capacity drive or work hardware. Drive or play out no sort of risky undertakings assuming naltrexone causes you any wooziness or other perilous secondary effects.

You shouldn't utilize naltrexone on the off chance that you are adversely affected by the medication, any vehicle or any idle fixings in the drug. Let your primary care physician know if you have at any point had a hypersensitive response to this medication or some other substance.

In the event that you are pregnant, breastfeeding or arranging a pregnancy, make certain to tell your PCP before you start naltrexone treatment.

Is naltrexone equivalent to naloxone?

No. Be mindful so as not to confound the name naltrexone with naloxone (brand name models: Narcan, Evzio).

Naloxone is utilized in a crisis narcotic excess to switch impacts like eased back or quit relaxing.

Naloxone isn't utilized in that frame of mind of narcotic use problem or liquor use jumble.

Are there drug cooperation with naltrexone?

There is the chance of a wide range of medication connections with naltrexone. You shouldn't begin taking any new physician endorsed medication, over-the-counter (OTC) prescription, nutrient, home grown or dietary enhancement until you have had a medication connection survey finished by your PCP or drug specialist.

Naltrexone will likewise obstruct the impacts of other narcotic containing meds, like hack and cold cures and antidiarrheal arrangements. While taking naltrexone, you may not profit from these drugs or narcotic analgesics. Continuously utilize a non-opiate medication to treat torment, the runs, or a hack. Get some information about the best medication to utilize.

Do I want a naltrexone distinguishing proof card?

Indeed, convey your naltrexone ID card with you consistently.

You ought to convey distinguishing proof to caution clinical faculty that you are taking naltrexone.

A naltrexone medicine card might be gotten from your PCP and guarantee that you can get sufficient treatment in a crisis.

Assuming you require clinical treatment, make certain to tell the treating doctor that you are getting naltrexone treatment.

The naltrexone infusion might cause an unfavorably susceptible kind of pneumonia. Patients ought to quickly advise their doctor assuming they foster signs and side effects of pneumonia, including inconvenience breathing, windedness, hacking, or wheezing.

Would it be a good idea for me to take naltrexone in the first part of the day or around evening time?

Most patients take their naltrexone tablet in the first part of the day, however the maker doesn't determine a specific time.

A few patients feel taking naltrexone toward the beginning of the day after breakfast is a decent indication of their proceeded with treatment responsibility for narcotic use problem or liquor use jumble.

Taking with food or a dinner might assist with bringing down sickness or stomach torment on the off chance that you experience this incidental effect.

In the event that your primary care physician has encouraged you to take naltrexone at a specific time or night, adhere to their directions all things considered.

Naltrexone ought to just be given as a component of a restoratively regulated enslavement treatment plan.

Naltrexone tablets might create problems with dozing (sleep deprivation) in around 3% (3 out of each and every 100) individuals who take it. It has likewise been accounted for to cause apprehension (4%) and uneasiness (2%). On the off chance that these are secondary affects you are encountering, talk with your primary care physician to decide whether taking your prescription in the morning may be useful.

Naltrexone may likewise prompt sleepiness, weariness or discombobulation and influence your capacity to drive or work apparatus. Play out no sort of risky errand assuming naltrexone influences you like this.

How long do I utilize naltrexone?

On the off chance that you are involving naltrexone tablets for liquor use jumble, your primary care physician might recommend this treatment for a considerable length of time or longer. Concentrates on led by the maker evaluated security and adequacy as long as 12 weeks. Try not to take additional pills, skip pills or stop your medicine until you converse with your PCP.

Elective tablet treatment regimens, other than one tablet consistently, might be utilized for support treatment for both liquor use jumble and narcotic use problem. Follow your physician's instruction for dosing.

On the off chance that you get the long-acting intramuscular infusion type of naltrexone (brand name: Vivitrol), you will just accept your infusion at your PCP's office one time each month. You don't give this prescription to yourself. The infusion will be delivered straightforwardly to your primary care physician. Try not to endeavor to provide yourself with an infusion of naltrexone. Injectable naltrexone has been related with serious infusion site responses and skin responses.

The period of time you will get naltrexone treatment is subject to your reaction to treatment and your objectives. Numerous patients get naltrexone infusion for somewhere around one year. Adhere to your PCP's guidance for dosing consistently.

Prior to beginning naltrexone, you should be without narcotic for at least 7 to 14 days to stay away from abrupt narcotic withdrawal. Patients who are truly subject to narcotics ought to finish detoxification before inception of naltrexone treatment.

Assuming that you ought to backslide after a time of narcotic forbearance, or stop naltrexone treatment, it is conceivable that the dose of narcotic that you recently utilized may have dangerous results, including respiratory capture (eased back or quit breathing), circulatory breakdown, and passing. Try not to utilize narcotics (opiates) with naltrexone.

How long does naltrexone function?

The 50-mg oral tablets have an impact that endures 24 to a day and a half. Higher portions have a more drawn out span, with 100 mg enduring 48 hours and 150 mg enduring 72 hours. Oral naltrexone tablets are generally allowed one time per day.

Blood levels of intramuscular naltrexone (brand name: Vivitrol) will start to gradually diminish 14 days subsequent to dosing, yet levels will be quantifiable for around one month.

Does naltrexone make you lethargic?

Tipsiness, sluggishness, sedation and swooning have all been accounted for as conceivable aftereffects with naltrexone treatment.

Try not to drive, work large equipment or play out some other hazardous exercises until you know what naltrexone will mean for you.

Naltrexone might make a few patients feel discouraged. Let your primary care physician know if you have a background marked by despondency, endeavored self-destruction, or other psychological wellness issues before you start naltrexone treatment. Tell your relatives or others near you that you are taking naltrexone. They ought to summon a specialist right in the event that you become discouraged or experience side effects of sorrow.

Main concern

The producer doesn't determine assuming you ought to take naltrexone tablets in the first part of the day or around evening time. Take naltrexone precisely as your primary care physician orders.

Numerous patients take their medicine in the first part of the day to assist with asserting their proceeded with treatment accomplishment for either narcotic use problem or liquor use jumble.

Taking naltrexone tablets with food or after a dinner might assist with decreasing any stomach secondary effects like sickness or torment.

Other Clinical Issues

The presence of other clinical issues might influence the utilization of this medication. Ensure you let your primary care physician know if you have some other clinical issues, particularly:

Misery, or history of or

Psychological sickness, or history of — Use with alert. May exacerbate these circumstances.

Bombed the naloxone challenge test (clinical trial to really take a look at your reliance to narcotic medication) or

Narcotic withdrawal, intense or

Positive pee test for narcotics or

Getting narcotic analgesics (eg, buprenorphine, methadone, morphine) — Ought not be utilized in patients with these circumstances.

Kidney illness or

Liver infection (counting cirrhosis, hepatitis B or C) — Use with alert. The impacts might be expanded in light of more slow expulsion of the medication from the body.

Appropriate Use

Take naltrexone consistently as requested by your PCP. It very well might be useful to have another person, like a relative, specialist, or medical caretaker, give you each portion as booked.

You should quit utilizing narcotics (opiates) for no less than 7 to 10 days before you can begin taking naltrexone. Your PCP might have to do the naloxone challenge test or a pee test for narcotics to ensure you are sans narcotic.

Dosing

The portion of this medication will be different for various patients. Follow your physician's instructions or the headings on the name. The accompanying data incorporates just the normal dosages of this medication. Assuming that your portion is unique, don't transform it except if your primary care physician instructs you to do as such.

How much medication that you take relies upon the strength of the medication. Additionally, the quantity of portions you require every day, the time permitted among dosages, and the period of time you take the medication rely upon the clinical issue for which you are utilizing the medication.

For oral measurement structure (tablets):

For liquor addiction:

Grown-ups — 50 milligrams (mg) one time each day.

Kids — Use and portion not set in stone by your PCP.

For opiate fixation:

Grown-ups — from the beginning, 25 milligrams (mg) (one-half tablet) for the principal portion, then, at that point, another 25 mg 1 hour after the fact. From that point onward, the portion is 350 mg each week. Your PCP will guide you to split this week by week portion and take naltrexone as per one of the accompanying timetables:

50 mg (one tablet) consistently; or

50 mg daily during the week and 100 mg (two tablets) on Saturday; or

100 mg each and every other day; or

150 mg like clockwork.

Youngsters — Use and portion not set in stone by your PCP.

Missed Portion

In the event that you miss a portion of this medication, accept it quickly. In any case, assuming it is nearly time for your next portion, avoid the missed portion and return to your standard dosing plan. Don't twofold portions.

Capacity

Store the medication in a shut holder at room temperature, away from intensity, dampness, and direct light. Hold back from freezing.

Keep out of the span of kids.

Try not to keep obsolete medication or medication at this point not required.

Ask your medical services proficient how you ought to discard any medication you don't utilize.

Safety measures

Your primary care physician genuinely must really look at your advancement at normal visits. Your primary care physician might believe that should do specific blood tests to check whether the medication is causing undesirable impacts.

This medication obstructs the "high" feeling you get from opiate (narcotic) drugs, including heroin. Since naltrexone might make you more delicate to bring down dosages of narcotics than you have recently utilized, you shouldn't utilize heroin or some other opiate medications to conquer what the medication is doing. You could go too far and foster difficult issues.

This medication might create difficult issues with your liver. Summon your primary care physician right on the off chance that you begin having dull pee, torment in the upper stomach, or yellowing of the eyes or skin while you are utilizing this medication.

This medication might expand considerations of self-destruction. Tell your PCP immediately in the event that you begin to feel more discouraged. Likewise tell your primary care physician immediately assuming you have considerations about harming yourself. Report any surprising considerations or ways of behaving that inconvenience you, particularly assuming they are new or deteriorate rapidly. Ensure your guardian knows whether you feel tired constantly, rest significantly more or much not exactly expected, feel sad or defenseless, or on the other hand in the event that you experience difficulty dozing, blow up effectively, have a major expansion in energy, or begin to act careless. Additionally, let your PCP know if you have unexpected or unmistakable inclinations, for example, feeling anxious, irate, fretful, fierce, or terrified.

Recall that utilization of naltrexone is just important for your treatment. Be certain that you follow your PCP's all's requests, including seeing your specialist as well as going to help bunch gatherings consistently.

Try not to attempt to conquer the impacts of naltrexone by taking opiates. To in all actuality do so may cause trance like state or passing. You might be more delicate with the impacts of opiates than you were prior to starting naltrexone treatment.

Naltrexone likewise obstructs the valuable impacts of opiates. Continuously utilize a non-opiate medication to treat torment, loose bowels, or a hack. Assuming you have any inquiries regarding the appropriate medication to utilize, check with your PCP.

Naltrexone won't keep you from becoming weakened when you drink liquor. Try not to take naltrexone to drive or perform different exercises while affected by liquor.

This medication might make certain individuals become dazed, sleepy, or less ready than they are regularly. Assuming any of these aftereffects happen, don't drive, use machines, or do anything more that could be risky on the off chance that you are discombobulated or are not ready while you are taking naltrexone.

Never share this medication with any other individual, particularly somebody who is utilizing opiates. Naltrexone causes withdrawal side effects in individuals who are utilizing opiates.

Tell every clinical specialist, dental specialists, and drug specialists you go to that you are taking naltrexone.

It is suggested that you convey recognizable proof expressing that you are taking naltrexone. Distinguishing proof cards might be accessible from your PCP.

Secondary effects

Alongside its required impacts, a medication might cause a few undesirable impacts. Albeit not these aftereffects might happen, on the off chance that they truly do happen they might require clinical consideration.

Check with your PCP right away assuming any of the accompanying secondary effects happen:

More uncommon

Skin rash

Interesting

Stomach or stomach torment (serious)

obscured vision, hurting, consuming, or enlarged eyes

chest torment

disarray

distress while peeing or incessant pee

fever

mind flights or seeing, hearing, or feeling things that are not there tingling

mental wretchedness or other state of mind or mental changes

ringing or humming in the ears

windedness

enlarging of the face, feet, or lower legs

weight gain

A few incidental effects might happen that normally don't require clinical consideration. These aftereffects might disappear during treatment as your body changes with the medication. Likewise, your medical care proficient might have the option to inform you concerning ways of forestalling or lessen a portion of these incidental effects. Check with your medical services proficient assuming any of the accompanying incidental effects proceed or are annoying or on the other hand in the event that you have any inquiries concerning them:

More normal

Stomach or stomach squeezing or torment (gentle or direct)

uneasiness, apprehension, fretfulness or inconvenience resting

cerebral pain

joint or muscle torment

queasiness or heaving

strange sluggishness

More uncommon

Chills

obstruction

hack, dryness, runny or stodgy nose, sinus issues, sniffling, or sore throat

loose bowels

discombobulation

quick or beating heartbeat

expanded thirst

peevishness

loss of craving

sexual issues in guys

What will occur assuming I drink liquor while taking naltrexone?

Naltrexone doesn't decrease the impacts of liquor that impede coordination and judgment. Naltrexone might decrease your sensation of inebriation and the craving to drink more, yet it won't make an extreme actual reaction drinking.

Is everything right to take different drugs with naltrexone?

You ought to convey a card (Structure C-6) making sense of that you might be on naltrexone, which trains clinical staff on torment the executives. Naltrexone doesn't diminish the adequacy of neighborhood and general sedation utilized with a medical procedure. Notwithstanding, it blocks help with discomfort from narcotic prescriptions. Many torment meds that are not sedatives are accessible. Assuming you are having elective medical procedure, you ought to quit taking naltrexone something like 72 hours in advance.

The significant dynamic impact of naltrexone is on sedative (opiate) drugs, which is one class of medications utilized fundamentally to treat torment but at the same time is tracked down in some solution hack arrangements. Naltrexone will obstruct the impact of typical dosages of this sort of medication. There are numerous nonnarcotic pain killers you can use while on naltrexone.

In any case, naltrexone is probably going to littly affect different prescriptions you may generally utilize like anti-infection agents, nonopioid pain relievers (e.g., headache medicine, acetaminophen/Tylenol®, ibuprofen/Motrin®/Advil®), and sensitivity drugs. You ought to illuminate your clinical clinician regarding the prescription you are right now taking so potential associations can be assessed.

Since the liver separates naltrexone, different drugs that can influence liver capability might influence the portion of naltrexone.

What will occur in the event that I become pregnant while taking naltrexone?

In the event that you have the organic potential to have a kid, you ought to utilize a powerful technique for contraception while taking naltrexone. Nonetheless, in the event that you miss a feminine period, report this to your clinical clinician immediately and take a pregnancy test. In the event that you become pregnant, you will cease the drug. Your clinical clinician ought to keep on getting some information about your wellbeing all through your pregnancy and furthermore about the soundness of your child after conveyance.

Would it be a good idea for me to take naltrexone with a feast?

There is no data that taking naltrexone regardless of feasts has any effect basically.

What occurs in the event that I quit taking naltrexone out of nowhere?

Naltrexone doesn't cause actual reliance, and you can quit taking it whenever without encountering withdrawal side effects.

Assuming I take naltrexone, does it imply that I don't require other treatment for liquor reliance?

No. Research studies have shown that naltrexone was best when it was joined with treatment from experts or potentially shared help gatherings.

What is the relationship of naltrexone to AA and other shared help gatherings?

There is no inconsistency between partaking in help gatherings and taking naltrexone. As a matter of fact, one multisite study showed that naltrexone-taking subjects who went to common care groups, like AA, had improved results. It is probably going to be powerful for you assuming you want to quit drinking through and through. Assuming other shared help bunch individuals alert against taking any meds, you ought to allude them to the flyer "The AA Part — Meds and Different Medications," which expressly expresses that AA individuals shouldn't "play specialist" and prompt others taking drugs given by genuine, informed clinical professionals or treatment programs.

Made in the USA
Coppell, TX
05 March 2024